Navigating Alzheimer's Disease

A FAMILY CAREGIVER'S GUIDE

BY
DR. DIANE DARBY BEACH,
GERONTOLOGIST

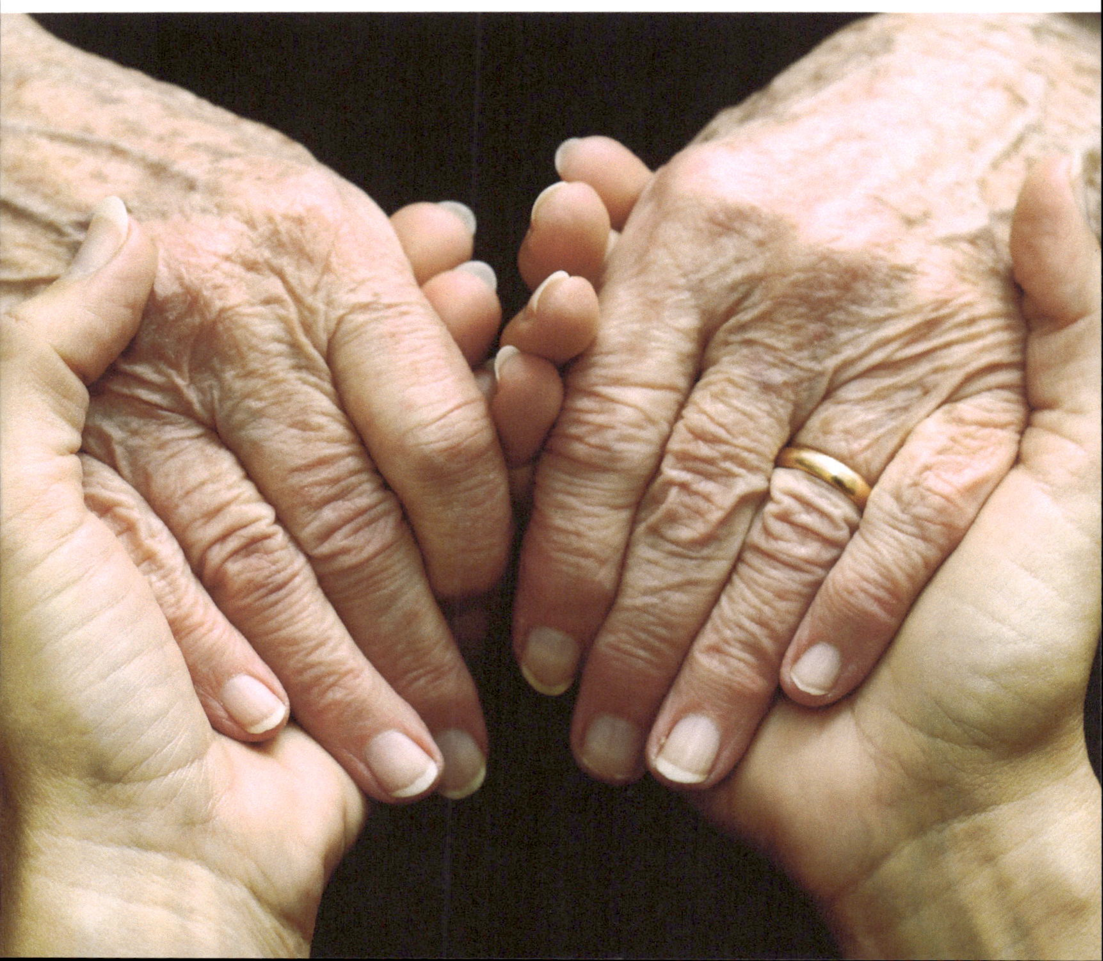

NAVIGATING ALZHEIMER'S DISEASE

©2018, DR. DIANE DARBY BEACH

All rights reserved. This book or any portion thereof may not be reproduced or used in any manner whatsoever without the express written permission of the author except for the use of brief quotations in a book review. Book design and layout by Susan Connell.

Printed in the United States of America

First Printing, 2018 ISBN 978-1973978022

CONTENTS

Foreword	i
Preface	ii
Is it Normal Memory Loss or Alzheimer's?	1
Caregiver Stress	5
What About the Kids?	9
Communication and Alzheimer's	13
Care Options	17
Hospice Service and Alzheimer's	23
The Financial Toll of Alzheimer's	27
Preventing Alzheimer's	33
Parting Comments	39
About the Author	40

FOREWORD

This handbook was written for caregivers and other loved ones watching someone very special to them suffer the journey of Alzheimer's disease. As family members and friends, we want our loved one to suffer little and yet the task of providing care can be daunting when we are already feeling overwhelmed. This handbook is intended to give you the basics of Alzheimer's and the detailed steps you will need to take while navigating this phase of your life. Believe it or not, the caregiving experience does not have to be entirely negative. In fact, when planned for, there are actually some beautiful moments along the way. Each chapter begins with information on the topic, followed by specific actions steps to be taken regarding that specific content area. My wish for you is a successful caregiving career; one most of you did not chose, yet lovingly embraced. I commend you for the task you have taken upon yourselves!

PREFACE

Being a caregiver to a loved one with Alzheimer's is the toughest job in the world. While you are providing 24/7 care and support, you are also grieving the loss of this person and the relationship you once had. You, of all people, do not have the time to read a long, detailed book on the do's and don'ts of caregiving. This handbook was written with you in mind. I hope you are able to gather information and helpful tips on key caregiver issues in a short, succinct manner.

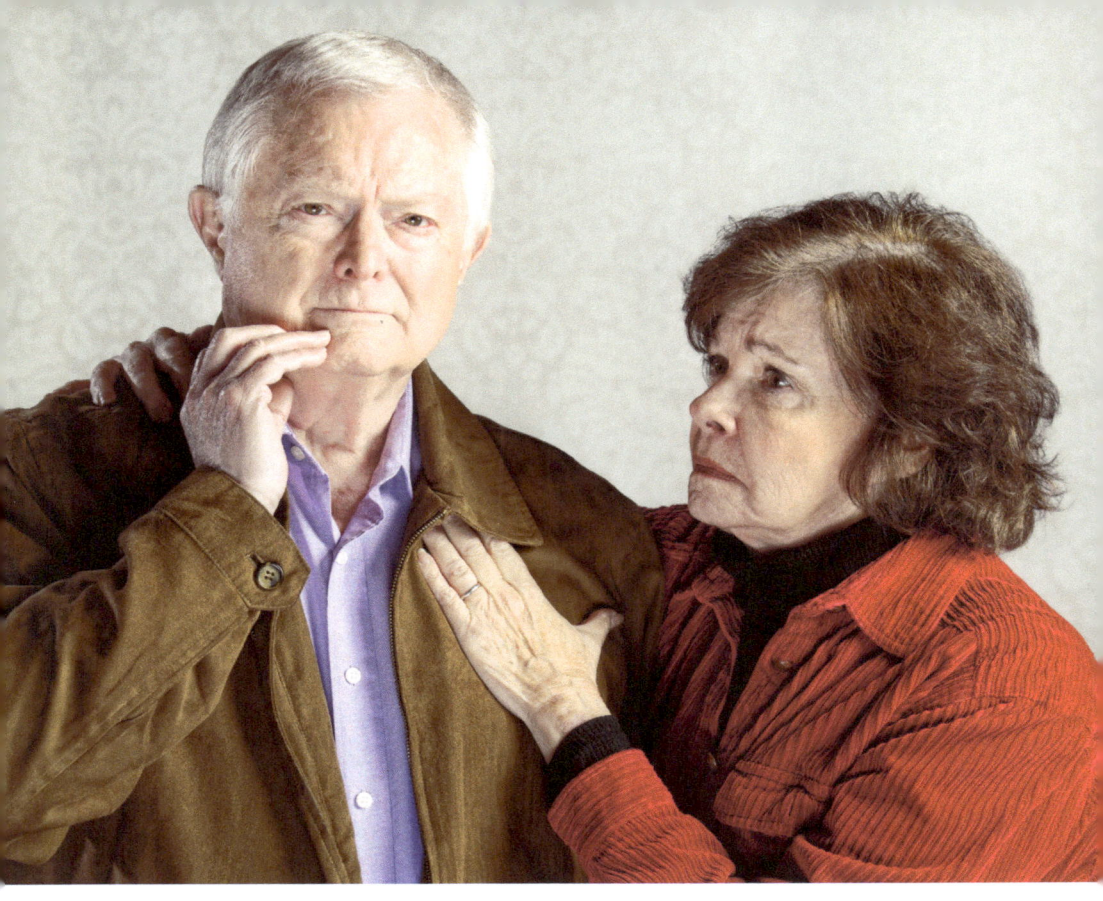

CHAPTER 1
IS IT NORMAL MEMORY LOSS OR ALZHEIMER'S?

Are you worried about the memory of someone you love? There is a difference between "normal" memory lapses and something more serious like Alzheimer's disease. It is important to recognize that Alzheimer's is more than just memory loss. Alzheimer's disease is a progressive, degenerative disease and many different parts of the brain are impacted, not just the brain's "memory banks." If you are concerned, take a look at the following 10 warning signs. If your loved one has two or more of the following, a visit to the doctor for a complete diagnostic work-up should be considered. An early as possible diagnosis is imperative as the medications used to treat the symptoms are best in the early to moderate stages of the disease. Don't wait!

THE 10 SYMPTOMS OF ALZHEIMER'S DISEASE:

1. Memory changes that disrupt daily life (can't remember parts of the morning routine such as brushing teeth or getting dressed).
2. Challenges in planning or solving problems (can't remember appointments).
3. Difficulty completing familiar tasks at home, at work, or at leisure (can't remember how to cook a meal or how to balance the checkbook).
4. Confusion with time or place (your loved one goes out to the grocery store, but is gone for three hours as he/she gets lost).
5. Trouble understanding visual images and spatial relationships (can't judge how far or close an object is or has trouble reading).
6. New problems with words in speaking or writing (uses "gibberish" words or has illegible writing).
7. Misplaces items and loses the ability to retrace steps (forgets why he/she walked in a room, but cannot retrace steps to recover the memory).
8. Decreased or poor judgment (starts giving money away to telephone solicitors or dresses for summer in the middle of December).
9. Withdrawal from work or social activities (your loved one with Alzheimer's may become depressed and refuse participation in everyday activities).
10. Changes in mood and personality (a very sweet person may become combative or vice versa).

ACTION STEPS:

If your loved one has two or more of the symptoms listed above, obtaining a proper diagnosis as soon as possible is vital! An appropriate diagnosis is much more than a simple 12-15-minute visit with your Primary Care Physician. A thorough diagnosis should be done by a Neurologist or a Geriatrician (a Doctor specializing in the treatment of older adults). Once this appointment is made, here's what to do:

- Write down all of the symptoms you have noticed about your loved one and bring this to the visit to discuss with the Doctor.
- Ask for blood work to be done (rules out metabolic problems, medication interaction issues and vitamin B-12 deficiency).If no issues show up in the blood work, ask for a CT scan and/or an MRI (this will rule out a brain tumor or a stroke).
- Finally, if these previous tests prove inconclusive, request a PT scan (this reveals the change of glucose metabolism in the brain associated with Alzheimer's disease).
- Once a diagnosis is made, ask the Doctor about the various symptom modifying medications that may be appropriate for your loved one. These include:
    1. Aricept
    2. Exelon
    3. Razadyne
    4. Namenda

Remember, these medications only modify symptoms. They do not cure the disease.

INSPIRATION

Acceptance is not submission; it is acknowledgement of the facts of a situation. Then deciding what you're going to do about it.

-Kathleen Casey Theisen

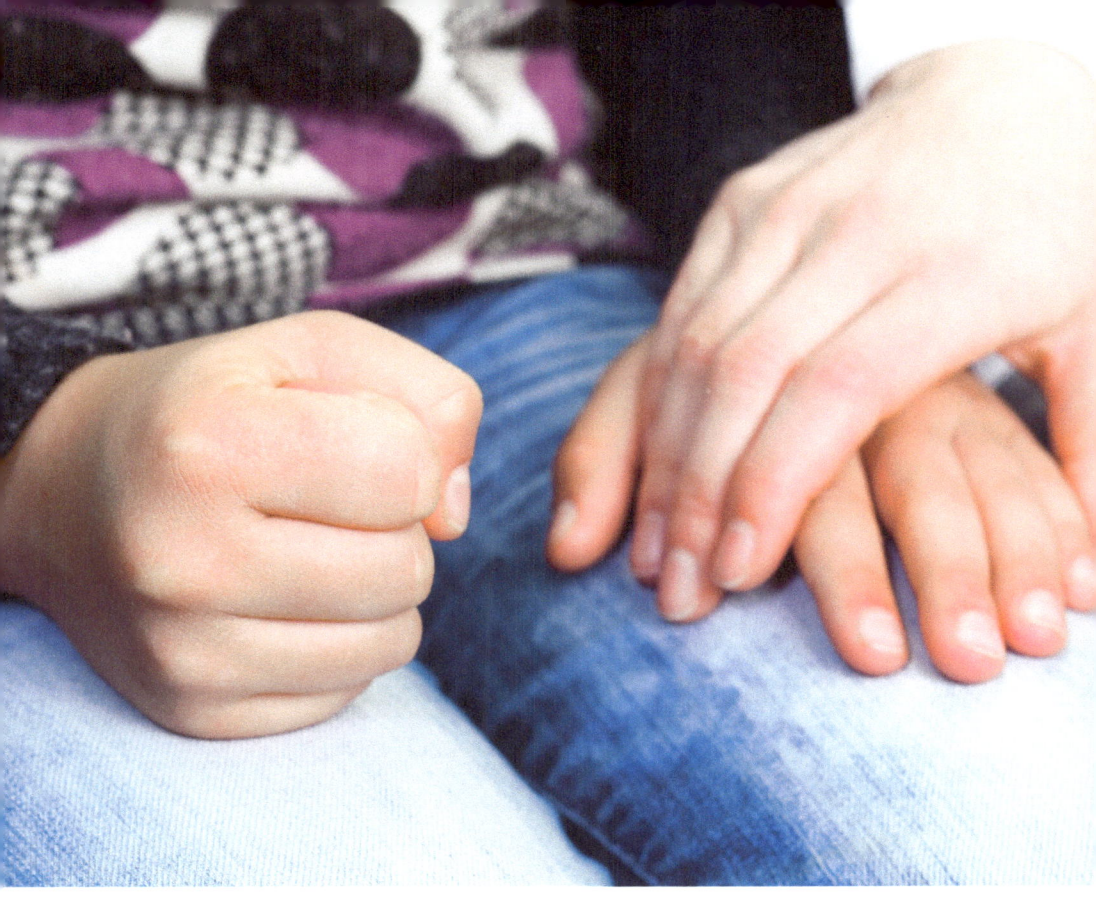

CHAPTER 2
CAREGIVER STRESS

Seventy percent of people with Alzheimer's disease are taken care of for the entirety of their disease by family caregivers. The responsibilities and challenges that come with caregiving can be overwhelming and stressful. Research in this area shows that between 40 and 70 percent of caregivers are significantly stressed and/or depressed. The symptoms of stress, burden, and depression can creep up on you with little notice of your condition. Once these symptoms set in, they can be extreme and persistent.

Symptoms of significant stress and depression include:

- Feelings of hopelessness or pessimism.

- Sad, anxious, or "empty" feelings.Loss of interest in once pleasurable hobbies or activities, including sex.
- Irritability, restlessness and anxiety.Feelings of guilt, worthlessness or helplessness.
- Persistent aches or pains, headaches, cramps, or digestive problems that do not ease, even with treatment.
- Overeating or appetite loss.
- Fatigue and decreased energy.
- Difficulty concentrating, remembering details, and making decisions.Insomnia, waking up during the night, or excessive sleeping.
- Thoughts of suicide or suicide attempts.

When caring for your loved one with Alzheimer's, you may also encounter "ambiguous grief." Specifically, your loved one is "here" in body, yet absent from relationships and many aspects of daily living. As such, you are caring and simultaneously grieving. This process creates yet another level of stress which can lead to depression.

Recognizing depression and stress is the first step to preventing it.

ACTION STEPS

Here some other things you can do to prevent these symptoms:

1. Talk about your feelings, frustrations, and fears with family, friends or a mental health professional.
2. Recognize that you are not alone; attend a support group to vent and hear from others in similar situations.
3. Take time for yourself. Meet a friend for lunch, take a class, or participate in a hobby.

4. Exercise. Physical activity produces dopamine and endorphins. You will feel better.
5. Breathe. When you are feeling overwhelmed, take a "time out" and force yourself to take three deep breaths.

MANAGING STRESS DURING THE HOLIDAYS

The holiday season can cause even more stress for caregivers. In prior years, you may have joyfully anticipated and participated in the hustle and bustle of the holiday season (including shopping, attending parties, tree decorating, cooking, etc.) Now, however, you may just want the whole thing over with. The additional stress of family gatherings, gift buying, cooking, and other obligations can become cumbersome. How can you, as a caregiver, better cope with this stress?

ACTION STEPS

The following tips may help you get through (and even enjoy) your holiday season.

1. Consider alternative shopping methods. The Internet is a convenient way to shop for food and gifts without ever leaving home. You can also choose gifts from catalogs without leaving your house. Minimize the hassle of shopping!
2. Scale back on rituals and traditions. We often feel compelled to live up to past holiday traditions, but it doesn't have to be that way. Suggest that someone else host Thanksgiving, Hanukkah or Christmas dinner. A potluck is also a great idea — delegate friends and family to bring favorite dishes.
3. Practice moderation. There are many attractive options in front of us during the holidays such as alcohol, sweets and high-calorie foods. Enjoy, but do not

over-indulge. (You don't want the stress of feeling sick the next day.)

4. Practice flexibility. Be prepared for unexpected circumstances. Something may come up, and probably will, so what can you do? If you can, change the situation. If you can't, accept it and move on. You cannot control life no matter how planned out you believe you have things. Laugh … it's OK.

5. Exercise. Try to keep up on your regular exercise routine, or start one, during the holidays. Walking several times a week is a great way to stay in shape, and it is easy to do. There is also something about pounding the pavement that helps release frustrations and clears your head.

6. Take breaks. Spend time with friends and take part in hobbies and other enjoyable activities such as yoga, meditation, needlepoint, reading, spending a couple of hours away from the house at the library, coffeehouse, etc.

INSPIRATION

Self-care is not selfish. You cannot serve from an empty vessel.
— Eleanor Brownn

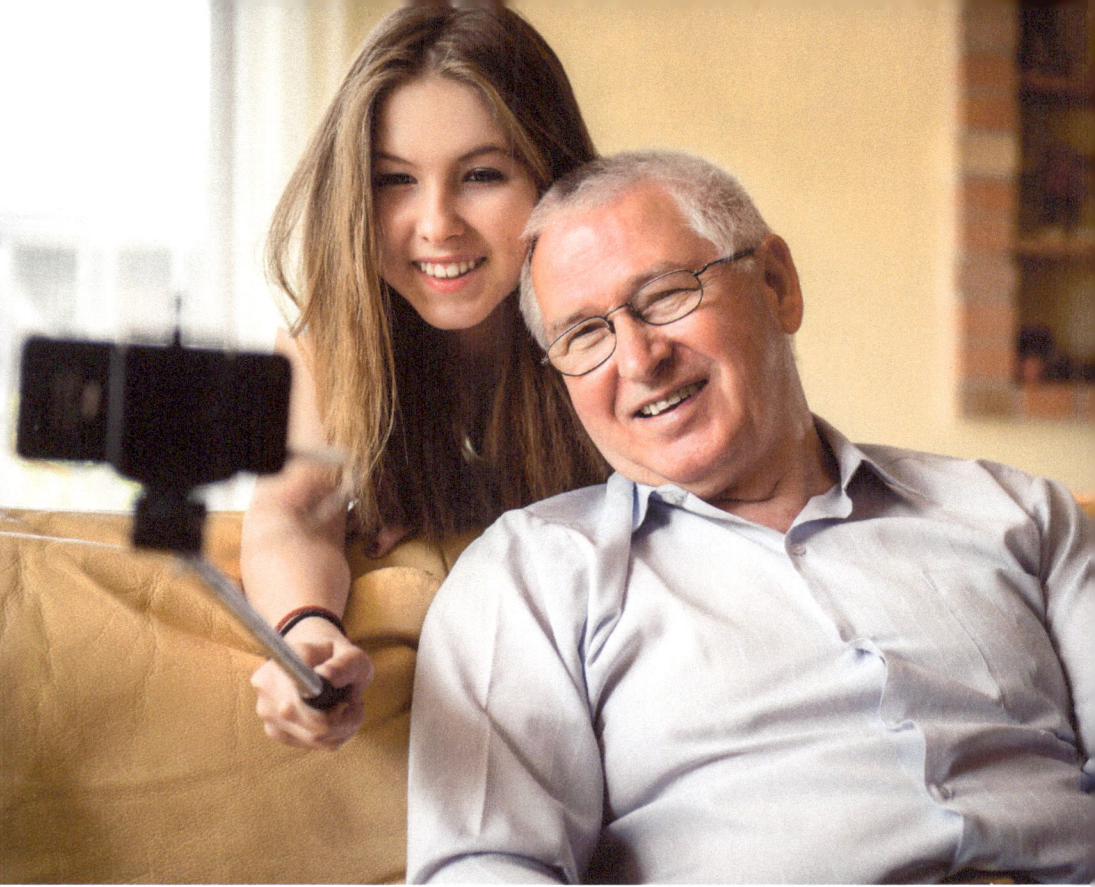

CHAPTER 3
WHAT ABOUT THE KIDS?

If you are an adult child caregiver, you may have children under the age of 18 living at home. You likely also work outside the home and may need to rely on your children to help with caregiving responsibilities. Research has shown that the caregiving experience as a younger person has both positive and negative outcomes.

Possible negative consequences for your pre-adolescent or adolescent caregivers follow:

- Peer relationships and social lives can be restricted, and as a result, your teen may feel isolated.
- Extracurricular activities and hobbies may be curtailed.

- Some are consistently late for school or absent altogether.
- The grandparent/grandchild relationship may suffer.
- If you, as the caregiver, are experiencing heavy stress, your pre-adolescent or teen is more likely to have more anxiety as well.
- These young caregivers may feel neglected by you, the parent caregiver, as so much attention is needed by your loved one with the disease.

Encouragingly, positive consequences for your young caregivers include:

- Your teen or pre-teen caregiver may grow closer to, and more protective of you, the caregiving parent.
- He/she may spend more quality time with his/her siblings.
- A younger caregiver may learn to be more patient with his/her grandparent and more flexible with the ever-changing family situation.
- He/she may be more selective of friends with the intention of protecting your loved one from any potential mocking or abuse by peers.

ACTION STEPS

1. Encourage your child to continue participation in activities such as hobbies, spending time with friends, engaging in sports, etc.

2. Talk openly with your child about the situation. Ask, "How are you feeling about this? Do we need to make any changes in the caregiving?"

3. Prompt your child to try and identify some positive points about the situation. For example ask, "Do you feel any closer to Grandma now that she lives with us?"

4. Make special "dates" with your child. Go to a movie, hit the gym together, get out for a meal. Try to schedule private time (without the loved one with the disease) each week. This will help prevent feelings of neglect/abandonment on your child's part.

5. Make sure you take time for yourself and manage your stress. The more stressed out you are, the more anxiety your child will experience.

> **INSPIRATION**
>
> Grief is the last act of love we have to give to those we loved. Where there is deep grief, there was great love.
>
> — Unknown

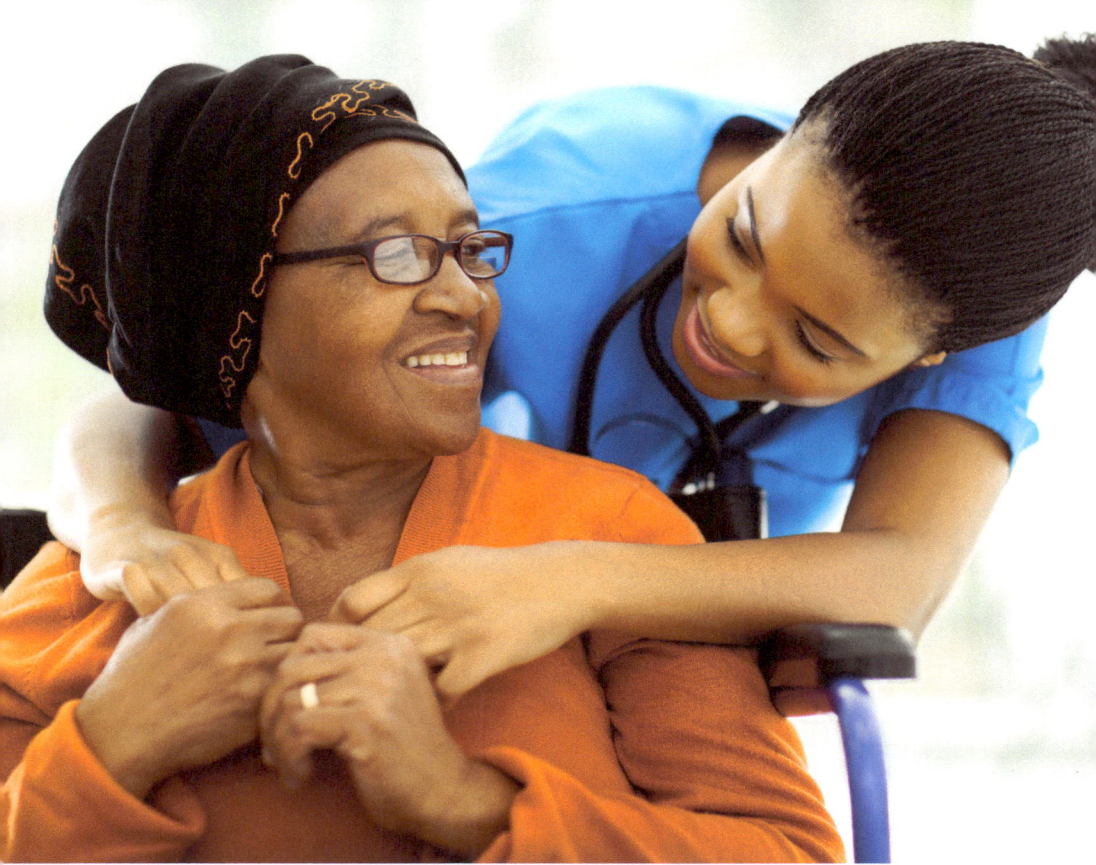

CHAPTER 4
COMMUNICATION AND ALZHEIMER'S

Losing the ability to verbally communicate can be one of the most frustrating and difficult issues for people with Alzheimer's disease, their families, and caregivers. The person with Alzheimer's experiences a gradual decline in the ability to communicate, finding it increasingly difficult to understand others and to clearly convey what he/she needs.

Each person with Alzheimer's is unique; there is no one-size-fits-all approach, and as such, strategies for communicating are unique to each person.

Symptoms of the disease progress differently for each person, affecting the brain in different ways. As a consequence, communication challenges will vary.

POSSIBLE COMMUNICATION CHALLENGES

- Your loved one may have difficulty finding a word. A related or non-sensical word might be uttered instead of the one not remembered.
- Your loved one may lose the ability to follow or join in a conversation or may fail to respond when spoken to.
- He/she may not be able to understand what you are saying or only comprehend part of it.
- He/she may use full sentences and familiar words, but not make sense.
- Writing skills may diminish/deteriorate.
- Reading skills may diminish/deteriorate.
- Emotions may be inappropriately expressed.

It is important to know that while your loved one's verbal skills are deteriorating, nonverbal communication skills are still very much intact. Interestingly, communication is 70 percent nonverbal and includes our body language, our facial expressions, our posture/gestures and the tone of our voice. Any negative nonverbal communication you display — such as sighing or frowning — can be easily picked up by your loved one and start a negative behavior cycle.

ACTION STEPS: COMMUNICATION DO'S

1. Speak in a gentle, caring manner. Keep sentences short and simple, giving instructions one step at a time.

2. Allow ample time for what you have said to be understood and for him/her to respond. Fill in words when needed.

3. Try to avoid over-stimulation via the TV, computer or radio.

4. Maintain regular routines which help reduce agitation and confusion.

5. Re-frame your perceptions in a positive light by emphasizing what your loved one CAN do; not what he/she can't do.

INSPIRATION

If you learn to listen for clues as to how I feel instead of what I say, you will be able to understand me much better.

— Mara Botonis

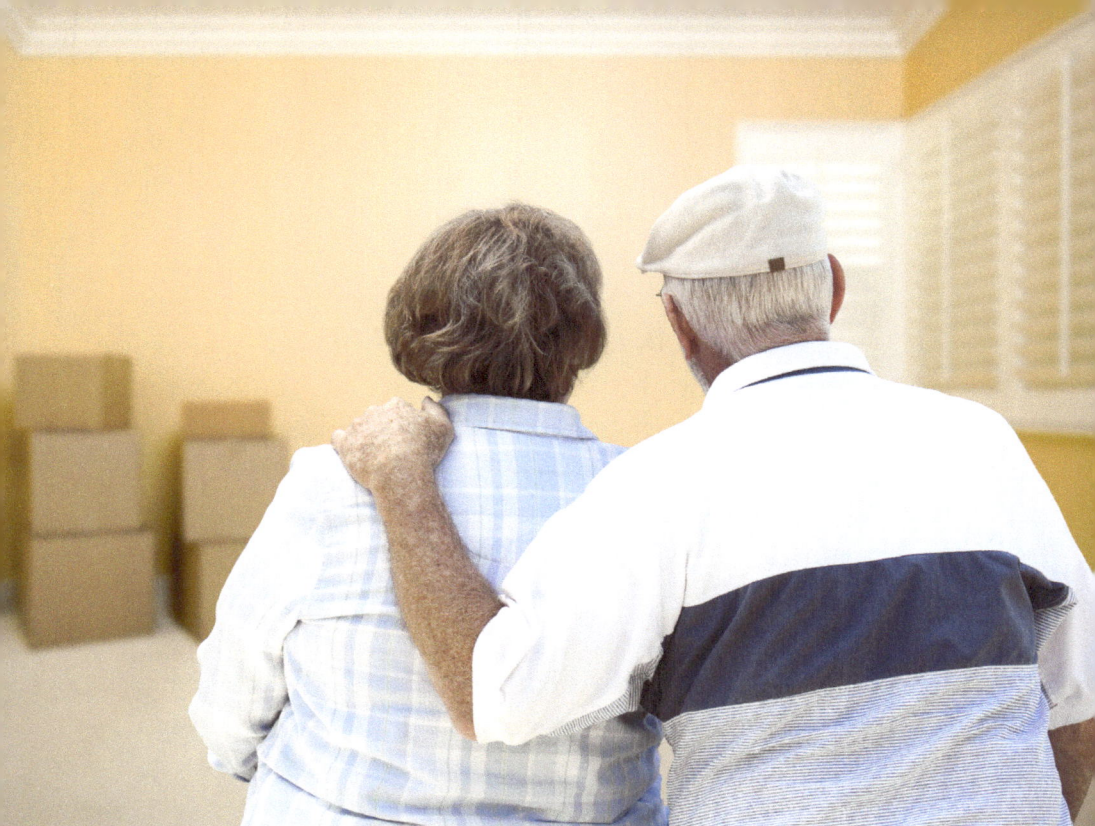

CHAPTER 5
CARE OPTIONS

Most of us want to stay in our own homes for as long as we can and we also wish this for our aging family members. Unfortunately, remaining at home alone is sometimes more dangerous to all involved.

So, when is the right time to make changes? How do we broach this sensitive subject with our loved ones? How do we convince ourselves (and our loved ones) that transitioning from the traditional home environment could actually be a better option?

None of us makes the best decisions when in crisis. So, waiting for your loved one to have a dangerous event before you consider care options is not optimal. Making decisions about when to arrange for care, where to find it and how to continue to keep up with changing needs, can be stressful and overwhelming. However, making some decisions about future care will likely lessen your worry about it in the future. Educate yourself on the options and start interviewing various home care agencies, tour assisted living facilities and day care providers. Find what is available in your community and help yourself prepare for the inevitable changes your loved one will experience.

AT HOME

Caring for someone with Alzheimer's disease at home is usually where most families start. A home environment may be preferable if it provides the socialization, comfort, and security to keep the individual with the disease content and engaged. The presence of family and friends can be very important for quality of life. However, safety may become an issue and lack of stimulation may lead to apathy or depression. An in-home care agency could assist with providing additional support.

ADULT DAY CARE

If your loved one with Alzheimer's is living at home, there may come a time when adult day care is a good way to receive a break and provide stimulation to the person with Alzheimer's. Some may have only complete day programs or they may offer half-day care and overnight care as well.

ASSISTED LIVING FACILITY

Assisted living facilities may be an appropriate care option for people with Alzheimer's in the early and moderate stages (and in some cases, through the late stages of the disease). When the effects of Alzheimer's become severe and the individual is no longer able to make decisions, or stay safe when unsupervised, an assisted living environment for Alzheimer's care may be an appropriate choice.

SKILLED NURSING

When a person with Alzheimer's deteriorates to a point where they can no longer live alone at all and they need a high level of medical care, a nursing home may be the most appropriate place for him/her. Some examples of appropriate skilled nursing care include the necessity for assistance with an i.v. g-tube, tracheotomy, open wound, or ventilator; care usually provided by trained skilled nursing staff including registered nurses (RNs), certified nursing assistants (CNAs), or licensed vocational nurses (LVNs).

These options are designed to allow people with Alzheimer's disease to receive the care they need while still maintaining their quality of life for as long as possible.

ACTION STEPS: TALKING WITH YOUR LOVED ONES

1. Plant the seed. Don't approach your loved one or other family members as though you've already made the decision for him or her. Count on broaching the subject several times (not just once). Ask a trusted friend in that person's life to also bring up the possibility of having an added level of care. Sometimes, this news is better received from someone outside the family.

2. Watch for a learning opportunity. For example, did Dad recently experience a fall, just missing a significant injury? Use this as a catalyst. After a recovery period, say something like, "That was a close call, maybe we could go have lunch at that new assisted living community close to home. It would be safer to have people around."

3. Check with your friends and friends of your loved ones. See if any are content using home care, adult day care or living in an assisted living community nearby, or if their parents are. Your aging family member might feel more comfortable if there were a friend already using extra care.

4. Tour more than one community and ask your loved one for feedback. Would they prefer a large community with lots of activities or a smaller, quieter board and care?

5. Stress your concern for their safety at home alone. If you are leaning towards moving your loved one to a community, emphasize the fact that there's no yard cleanup, but they can work in the garden when they want and there's no need to call a handyman when the house requires maintenance.

6. Lastly, be sensitive to your loves one's feelings. Bringing someone into the home or leaving a home where so much history has been conceived is not easy.

ACTION STEPS: WHAT TO LOOK FOR AMONG CARE OPTIONS

1. Staff speaking in a gentle, caring manner.
2. Staff keeping sentences short and simple, giving instructions one step at a time.
3. Staff allowing ample time for your loved one to understand and respond to what's been said. Fill in words when needed.
4. Staff avoiding over-stimulation via the TV, computer or radio.
5. Staff maintaining regular routines which help reduce agitation and confusion.

6. Staff maintaining their perceptions in a positive light by emphasizing what the person with Alzheimer's CAN do; not what he/she can't do.

INSPIRATION

With each new day I put away the past and discover the new beginnings I have been given.

— Angela L. Wozniak

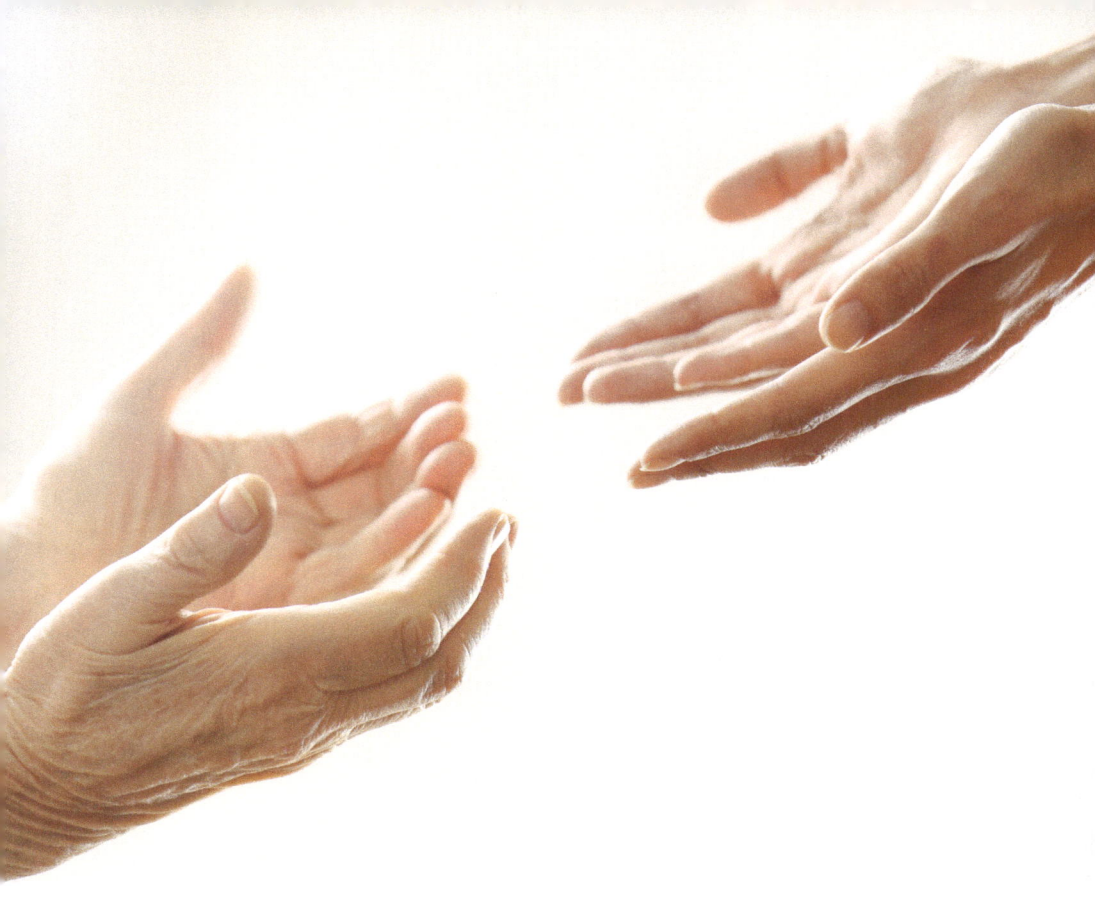

CHAPTER 6
HOSPICE SERVICE AND ALZHEIMER'S

Hospice Care is high-quality, compassionate care that can help your loved one and your entire family. Hospice is not "giving up," nor is it a form of euthanasia or physician-assisted suicide. Hospice serves those in the end stages of Alzheimer's disease by relieving pain, controlling symptoms, improving quality of life, and reducing anxiety and worry for you and your loved one. This type of care can be delivered in the your home, a long term care facility or an assisted living community.

The hospice team evaluates your loved one's status and updates the plan of care as symptoms and conditions change, even on a day-to-day basis. The goal of hospice is to relieve physical and emotional distress so that individuals retain their dignity and remain comfortable. As Alzheimer's disease progresses, your loved one may lose the ability to express his/her needs. Hospice will design a plan that addresses pain, hydration, nutrition, skin care, recurrent infection and agitation—all common problems associated with Alzheimer's.

ACTION STEPS

Look for these common signs that the disease has progressed to a point where all involved in the care of your loved one would likely benefit from hospice care:

1. Your loved one can say only a few words.
2. Your loved one can no longer walk and may be bedbound.
3. Your loved one is totally dependent on others for his/her activities of daily living such as: eating, dressing and grooming.
4. Your loved one shows signs of severe anxiety.
5. Your loved one becomes incontinent.
6. Your loved one has choking episodes or difficulty with breathing.
7. Your loved one has significant weight loss (>10% body weight in 6 months).

Ask your loved one's physician to make a recommendation for hospice services. Hospice can be ordered by a Physician based on his/her life expectancy and/or difficulty with activities of daily living.

> **INSPIRATION**
>
> Kindness is a language which the deaf can hear and the blind can see.
>
> — Mark Twain

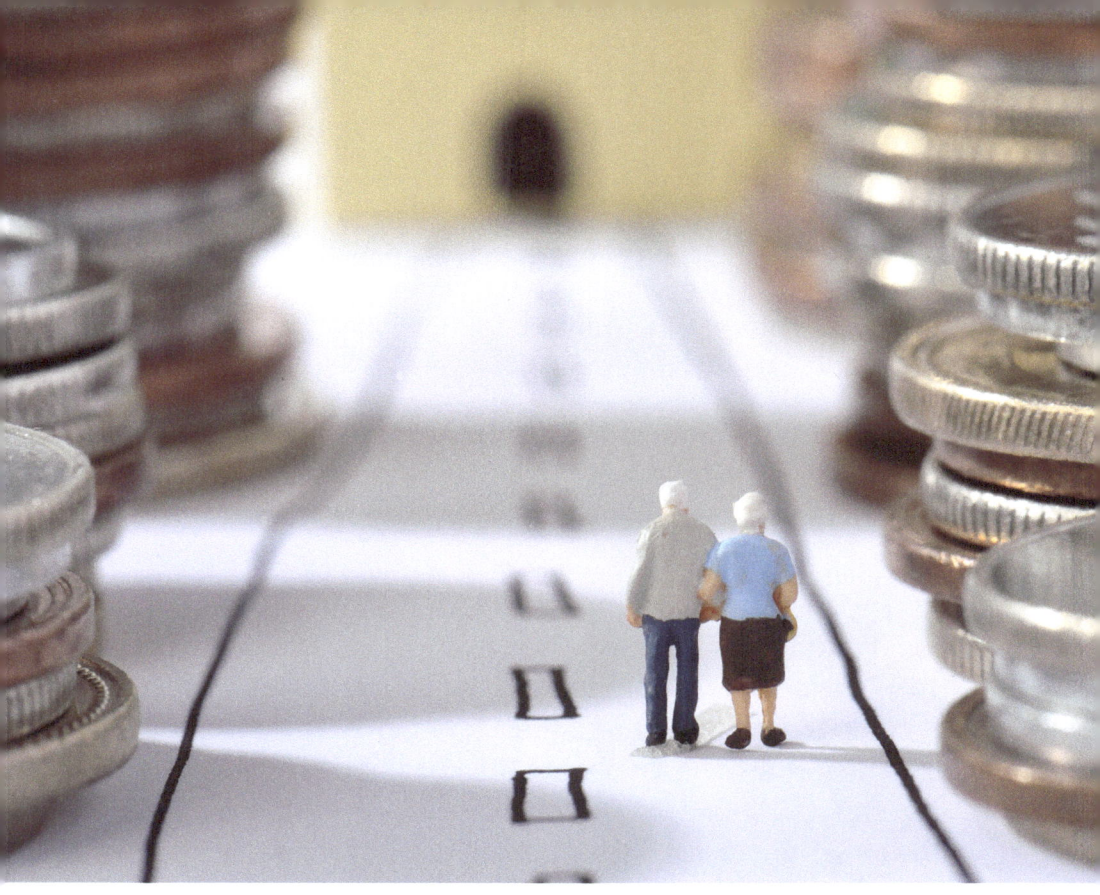

CHAPTER 7
THE FINANCIAL TOLL OF ALZHEIMER'S

An estimated 5 million people in the United States have Alzheimer's disease; this number is expected to double by the year 2050 as the elderly segment of our population grows. Specifically, as the Baby Boomers age, the incidence of Alzheimer's disease will increase. Not only does the disease have a significant emotional impact on individuals and their families, it can also cause severe family financial burden and places considerable demands on the greater public health system.

Most families take care of long-term care using these resources:

- Out of pocket
- Long-term care insurance
- Medicaid

While many long-term care insurance policies cover the level of care needed by an Alzheimer's patient, most people don't have such policies.

AT-HOME CAREGIVERS

Family and friends provide the majority of at-home care. On average, these families contribute an additional US$218 monthly toward the care of their loved one. This results in an annual contribution of more than $12,000, in addition to providing 24/7 care for that individual. Considering the fact that most individuals live with the disease for eight years (the range is two to 25 years), this financial burden can quickly compound into six-digit figures. Specifically, if an individual with the disease lives for eight years at home with full-time family caregiving, the bill would be $100,000. However, if the individual lives 15-20 years after diagnosis, the family will be faced with a financial toll ranging from $188,000-$250,000.

Given that the majority of care is done at home, many families are looking for part-time or full-time in-home assistance. These options include: home health aids, adult day care services, and adult day health care programs. These options range from $56 to $152 daily. For example, adult day care services average $68 per day, but can run from $25 to $100 a day. The average rate for an in-home health aid is $20 per hour.

MEDICARE

Many people falsely assume that Medicare will pay for long-term care needs. Unfortunately, Medicare pays for only a very small portion of these expenses. Recipients pay premiums entitling them to health services, limited home health care, and prescription drugs. Medicare also covers short stays in skilled nursing facilities when the need for admission immediately follows hospitalization for an acute illness (such as a heart attack or broken hip). Medicare will not subsidize on-going, long-term care in an assisted living community or nursing home.

MEDICAID

Medicaid (Medi-Cal in California), is a publicly funded program that funds health services for low-income or disabled Americans. The program obtains funds from both the federal government and individual states. Unlike Medicare, Medicaid covers basic health services and other long-term care services (including nursing home care). Unfortunately, to qualify for Medicaid, recipients must be considered "poor" or "indigent" by state standards. Fortunately, there are certain allowances for the well spouse, so assets can be somewhat protected.

COST OF CARE*

- On average, families contribute an additional $218 monthly toward the care of their loved one.
- The average hourly rate for an in-home health aid is $20 per hour. Adult day care services average $68 per day, but can range from $25 to $100 daily.

- The average cost for a private, one-bedroom unit in an assisted living facility is approximately $3,628 per month.
- The average cost for a private room in memory care is $5,100 per month.
- The average cost for a private, one-bedroom unit in a nursing home is $7,698 per month.

Genworth, Inc. (2016). Cost of Care Survey

PRIMARY SOURCES FOR LONG-TERM CARE FINANCING

Most families finance Alzheimer's care using multiple resources:

- 36% Out of pocket
- 20% Medicare
- 29% Medicaid (Medi-Cal)
- 5% Other (long-term care insurance)

ACTION STEPS

These statistics certainly give a grim snapshot of the financial toll Alzheimer's can take on your family. Plan ahead:

1. Decide how your loved one will be cared for at home, with adult day care, in an assisted living community, or in a nursing home.
2. It is imperative that you, your family (and the loved one, depending on the stage of the disease) start talking among yourselves, to other family members, and to professionals specializing in eldercare financial planning.
3. Prevent yourself from having to manage your finances in crisis mode to minimize the potential negative, lifelong impact on your family's financial health.

INSPIRATION

Everything has its wonders, even darkness and silence, and I learn, whatever state I may be in, therein to be content.
— Helen Keller

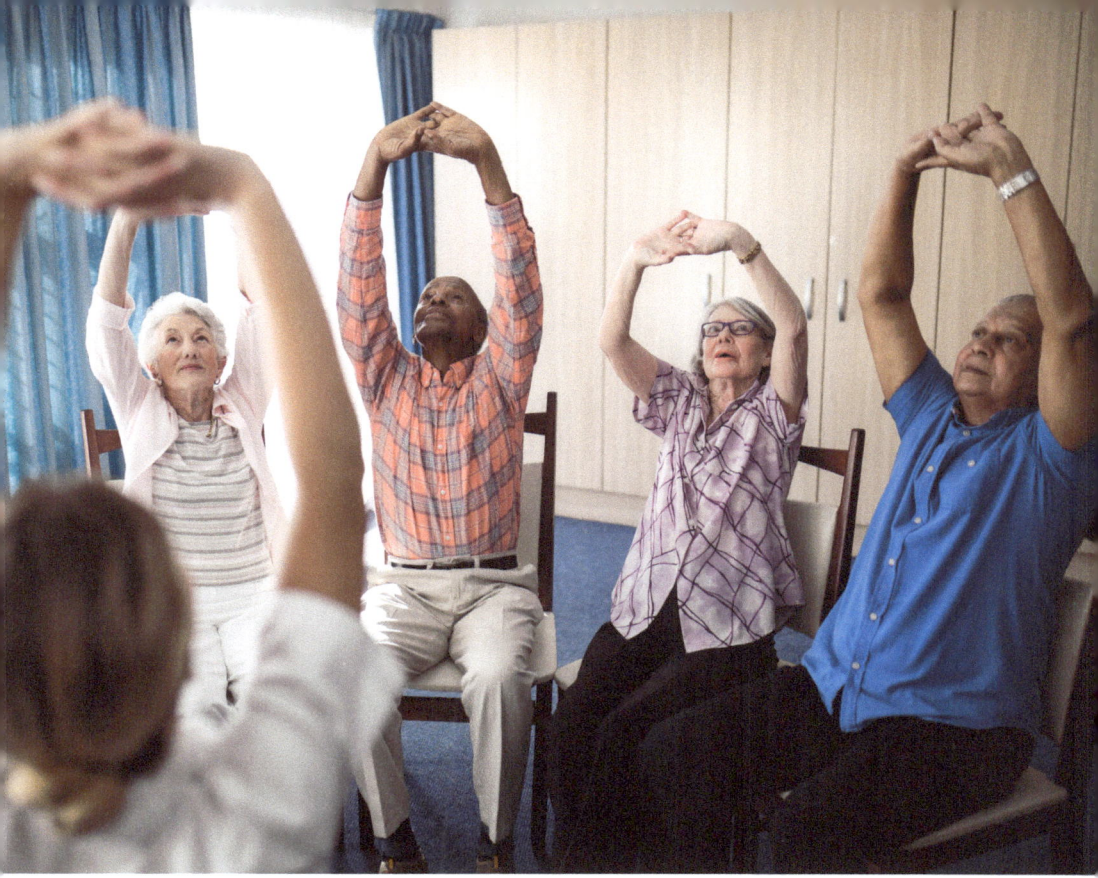

CHAPTER 8
PREVENTING ALZHEIMER'S

As we know the saying, "An ounce of prevention is worth a pound of cure." Is there anything you can do to prevent this from happening to you? The answer is this: You may not be able to completely eliminate the possibility of getting the disease, but you can reduce your risk significantly by living a "brain-healthy life." Recent research has linked certain lifestyle components to an increase in cognitive function and a decreased risk of developing Alzheimer's disease and other types of dementia. A brain-healthy lifestyle includes the following: physical exercise; mental exercise; sound nutrition; social connection; and avoidance of cardiovascular disease.

PHYSICAL EXERCISE: GET MOVING!

Research studies show that regular physical exercise (three to four times a week) may have significantly positive effects on brain function. Ideally, you want to aim for exercise sessions of moderate duration (30-40 minutes each). If you can combine cardio or aerobic exercise with strength and flexibility training, you'll get the greatest cognitive benefit. Some examples include: walking; tennis; jogging; swimming; strength training; yoga, tai chi; and dancing. You will be more successful at exercising if you do something that you like and something that is convenient. What does that mean?

ACTION STEPS

- Pick an activity that you enjoy! If you dislike walking, don't make it your goal to walk 4-5 times a week. You will give up after a few times.
- Choose an exercise class or gym that is convenient. Don't sign up for a gym or class that is 15 miles from where you live or 12 miles from work. You will be a lot less likely to make it to class!
- Make an exercise "date" with a family member or friend. This way, you are accountable and less likely to skip the workout!

EXERCISE YOUR BRAIN! IF YOU DON'T USE IT, YOU WILL LOSE IT!

Studies show that if we don't "exercise" our brains, we may actually lose brain function. For example, regular participation in activities that require higher levels of concentration or social interaction are associated with better cognitive function. In fact, people who engage in cognitively stimulating activities are less likely to be diagnosed with Alzheimer's disease. These types of activities actually stimulate new brain cell and neurotransmitter growth at any age. You can be 8, 18, 80, or 108 years old and still grow new brain cells!

ACTION STEPS

- Engage in leisure activities such as reading, playing board games, attending classes, or playing a musical instrument.
- Take a class at the local library or community center.
- Attend a local concert.
- Stay up with current events (read the newspaper).
- Join a book club.

YOU ARE WHAT YOU EAT!

Studies show promising results regarding nutrition and brain health. For example, there appears to be a direct correlation between vitamin E and risk reduction of Alzheimer's disease. In addition, research shows the benefits of vitamin C as a protective measure against the disease. The omega 3 fatty acids and deep, green leafy vegetables also provide protection.

ACTION STEPS

- Incorporate spinach, kale, broccoli, and brussels sprouts into your diet.
- Add strawberries, blueberries, raspberries, and prunes as snacks during the day.
- Munch on almonds, hazelnuts, and sunflower seeds, rather than potato chips.
- Consume salmon, mackerel, herring, tuna, and whitefish as lunch or dinner 2 times a week.

STAY CONNECTED

Social connection may also reduce the risk of developing Alzheimer's. People who isolate are at greater risk of depression, which has been repeatedly associated with Alzheimer's. As such, remaining involved with friends and family may protect you from the detrimental cycle of loneliness that often leads to cognitive dysfunction.

ACTION STEPS

- Call up a friend or family member you've lost touch with.
- Attend a class in the community.
- Start a hobby with a friend.
- Meet a friend for coffee.
- Have "game night" at your house and invite extended family and friends.

HEART HEALTH EQUALS BRAIN HEALTH

Cardiovascular disease has been linked to brain health. In other words, what is good for your heart is good for your brain! Researchers have documented that those of us with high systolic blood pressure (the top number) have a 2.3-fold greater risk of developing Alzheimer's disease. Moreover, individuals with low levels of HDL cholesterol (the good cholesterol) are more than twice as likely to develop cognitive decline compared with those who have high levels of this good kind of cholesterol.

ACTION STEPS

- Monitor your diabetes.
- Control your blood pressure.
- Reduce the bad type of cholesterol.
- Quit smoking.

INSPIRATION

You gain strength, courage, and confidence by every experience in which you really stop to look fear in the face. You must do the things which you think you cannot do.

— Eleanor Roosevelt

PARTING COMMENTS

I hope that this guidebook has given you information in a concise, useful manner. If you take away one piece of information from this reading, please remember to take care of yourself! You will only be helpful to your loved one if you are healthy and rested!

For more information, please visit my website: www.HelpMeWithMyParent.com

www.ingramcontent.com/pod-product-compliance
Lightning Source LLC
Chambersburg PA
CBHW040332220526
45473CB00009B/2662